The Qi Gong Diet

Nutrition and movement according to TCM

Qi Gong and Dietetics are part of Traditional Chinese Medicine (TCM). The goal of Qi Gong is to maintain the health of body and mind through movement, breathing and imagination, and thus to lead a long, happy life. Dietetics deals with the way food is consumed with the aim of using it to prevent and treat diseases. The holistic approach applies in each case, that physical and psychological aspects influence each other. Qi Gong and Dietetics also lead to weight reduction and an increase in performance.

The author has been teaching Kung Fu and Qi Gong at his own school for many years. He had previously learned both arts from European and Chinese masters. His Qi Gong books contain useful knowledge and practical instructions in a compact, easy-to-understand form. Jin means "today" and Dao means "the way".

The Qi Gong Diet, Nutrition and movement according to TCM
1st edition, August 2023
Copyright © Jin Dao 2023
Cover image: pixabay.com
Photos: Marlon
Production and publishing: BoD - Books on Demand, Norderstedt
ISBN: 978-3755757405

JIN DAO-Publishing
66424 Homburg
www.WT-Saarpfalz.de
E-Mail: Kontakt@WT-Saarpfalz.de

Content

Introduction

I have been teaching traditional Qi Gong for many years. In order to make the resulting experience and the exercises, some of which are thousands of years old, accessible to as many interested parties as possible, I have written a series of six practical volumes. These are titled "Stay young with Qi Gong!" and include standing, sitting, walking and lying exercises that are partly internal and partly external in nature. In this book I have only been able to reproduce a small selection of them, otherwise this would have gone beyond the scope. If required, you can find many more exercises and useful background knowledge in the volumes mentioned above.

According to Daoist teachings, Qi permeates everything in the universe – including people. Qi Gong therefore has many positive effects on our health and life. Among other things, regular exercise leads to an improvement in metabolic processes and the consumption of excess energy reserves, which in turn increases well-being and, in the case of overweight, leads to weight reduction.

The Qi naturally has a slow progression. Accordingly, Qi Gong exercises are always carried out slowly, calmly and carefully. The same applies to the time and duration in which we should devote ourselves to our practices. Working with Qi is not a sprint, athletic competition, wellness, or fad. Instead, you should permanently integrate simple exercises into your daily or weekly schedule. Even if you can often perceive the amazing energetic effect of Qi Gong after the first try, the best and most lasting successes will come over time.

A book about the state of our bodies would be incomplete without nutritional information and advice. Qi Gong is a part of traditional Chinese medicine, as is Dietetics - the teaching that deals with the effects and composition of individual foods. Another instrument that is now also gaining recognition in western medicine is the Organ (body) clock. This explains which organs are particularly active or inactive at which times.

With the knowledge imparted here, which we call the "Qi Gong diet", you will be able to make your first practical experiences with Qi Gong and, if necessary, make some additional diet-specific adjustments.

Some quotations from Laozi (Lao Tse), the founder of Daoism and author of the Daodejing (Tao Te Ching) from the 6th century BC:

"The mightiest thing in the world is that which cannot be seen, heard, or touched."

"Where there is much shadow, there must be much light hidden."

"The wise man has no indisputable principles. He adapts."

"You are not only responsible for what you do, but also for what you don't do."

"Those who dominate others are strong. He who controls himself is powerful."

"Desirelessness leads to inner peace."

"When you realize that you lack nothing, the whole world is yours."

"Those who smile instead of raving are always the stronger ones."

"The one who knows his goal will find the way."

What is Qi Gong?

Qi Gong (qigong) is one of the pillars of Traditional Chinese Medicine (TCM) alongside acupuncture, pharmaceutics, Dietetics and Tuina (massage). Its beginnings are around 10,000 BC supposed. Regular practice of Qi Gong has the objective of maintaining physical and mental health, or restoring it where necessary. Also, the body is said to be rejuvenated in general. As a result, the aim is to achieve longevity in connection with the best possible physical constitution. Daoism, Buddhism and the Asian martial arts have had a significant influence on the teaching.

Qi means "life force" or "life energy". According to Chinese scholars, Qi is the basis of all phenomena, the primal force of all life and non-life. The Far Eastern world view states that everything in the universe consists of Qi, i.e. subtle energy. It is not tied to any specific appearance that would limit it, but can assume different physical states, forms and modes of action as required. When it gathers, it manifests into solid matter. When it disperses, it takes on subtle forms. Qi is contained in inanimate things like fire or water, in plants like grass or trees, and of course in humans and animals. Where there is Qi, there is life. A stagnation or absence of Qi is therefore equivalent to death. In the midst of a world that is subject to constant change and change, the presence of Qi is the only constant.

Gong means "work", "skill" or "ability". *Qi Gong* could therefore be translated as "work with life energy".

The character for Qi commonly used in China today (see Figure 1) consists of two individual characters. Below is the sign for "rice" and above is the sign for "fly" or "evaporate".

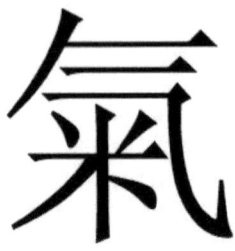

Figure 1

The Qi flows within the human being on the energy channels, the so-called *meridians*. If there is enough Qi in the body and it can flow freely, then the person is healthy. Otherwise, weaknesses and diseases can develop. Both external and internal factors can be considered as causes of a lack of Qi or a blockage of the free flow. External disease factors can be cold, heat, wind, humidity and drought. Internal disease factors are e.g. stress, overwork and long-lasting or suppressed feelings and emotions such as anger, joy, sadness, fear and worries. In addition, the way of life plays a major role, which should be characterized by a mindful and responsible treatment of oneself. Another danger comes from other factors, such as excesses, injuries, infections, etc. out of.

If a person feels ill, TCM believes that healing can be brought about by supporting the Qi in its work by practicing Qi Gong.

Qi Gong is a holistic concept that knows no separation between body, soul and spirit and always considers the entirety of all energetic processes. Instead of looking at certain symptoms and phenomena in isolation, Qi Gong activates the body's self-healing powers – the so-called "inner doctor" – so that it is able to regenerate itself if necessary.

The maintenance of health through the cultivation of Qi is thus the declared task of Qi Gong. This purpose is achieved in the following way:

1.Open the Qi Gong points (acupuncture points).
2.Lead fresh Qi into the body
3.Eliminate spent Qi (Xie Qi) from the body
4.Getting the Qi to flow
5.Eliminate Qi congestion and blockages (disharmonies).

The famous Daoist Ge Hong refers in his book "Baopuzi", which is datet back to around 300 AD, to the ubiquity of Qi:

"Man lives in the midst of Qi, and Qi fills man. From heaven and earth to the ten thousand beings, everything requires Qi to live. Anyone who knows how to manage the Qi nourishes his body on the inside and wards off harmful influences on the outside."

In the "Yellow Emperor's Classic on Internal Medicine" by Huang Di (probably 1st millennium BC), the standard work of traditional Chinese medicine, it says:

"The Qi of heaven nourishes the spirit of man, the Qi of earth nourishes his body. Both together bring about the activity of the entire organism."

The famous Swiss doctor and philosopher Theophrastus Bombast von Hohenheim, known as Paracelsus, wrote:

"He is a doctor who knows about the invisible, which has no name, no matter and yet its effect."

The positive effects of continuously performing Qi Gong exercises include the following:

-Strengthening of the immune system and self-healing powers
-Strengthening of the internal organs
-Increasing the elasticity of the fascia
-Dissolving blockages and tensions
-Relief of chronic ailments
-Slowing down the aging process
-Alertness and mental fitness into old age
-Feeling of freshness and inner strength
-Feeling of calm and serenity
-Reducing the need for sleep
-More positive charisma to our fellow human beings
-Increase in physical and mental flexibility
-Improved ability to spot opportunities and solve problems
-Increase in mental strength, resilience and performance
-Increase in self-confidence
-Higher quality of life and joie de vivre
-Faster recovery from injuries.

There is an almost unlimited number of individual Qi Gong exercises and about 100 conceptual types that are generally recognized. In order to get an overview of the different approaches and to structure them at least to some extent, one traditionally divides them into *internal* and *external* Qi Gong exercises.

The outer practices are called *Wai Dan* ("Outer Breath"). They include all methods that are primarily aimed at movement. It is therefore characteristic of Wai Dan exercises that the body is moved on the outside and relaxed on the inside. The inner practices are called *Nei Dan* ("Inner Breath"). Sometimes one also speaks of *Silent Qi Gong*. These include methods that trigger processes in the body and mind that are not visible from the outside, such as directing the Qi using the imagination, breathing exercises or the static assumption of certain postures. It is therefore characteristic of Nei Dan exercises that the body is moved internally and relaxed externally.

Qi Gong exercises must not be confused with sporting activities or relaxation techniques. In order for them to develop their holistic health benefits, they must have three elements in particular: awareness of the respective movement/posture, awareness of the direction and flow of energy (Qi) through imagination and awareness of breathing. In addition, relaxation, quiet, naturalness and leisurely pace are often mentioned as basic requirements.

Qi Gong exercise = movement + imagination + breathing

The Qi Gong principle = body (movement, posture) + mind (imagination - sometimes also called "heart") + breath

The Daoist philosopher Zhuangzi (Dschuang Chi) wrote in the 4th century BC:

"Inhale and exhale to take in the new and let go of the old, stretch like a bear and like a bird - this is Dao Yin (Qi Gong) to prolong life. This is how the sages practice when they practice this art."

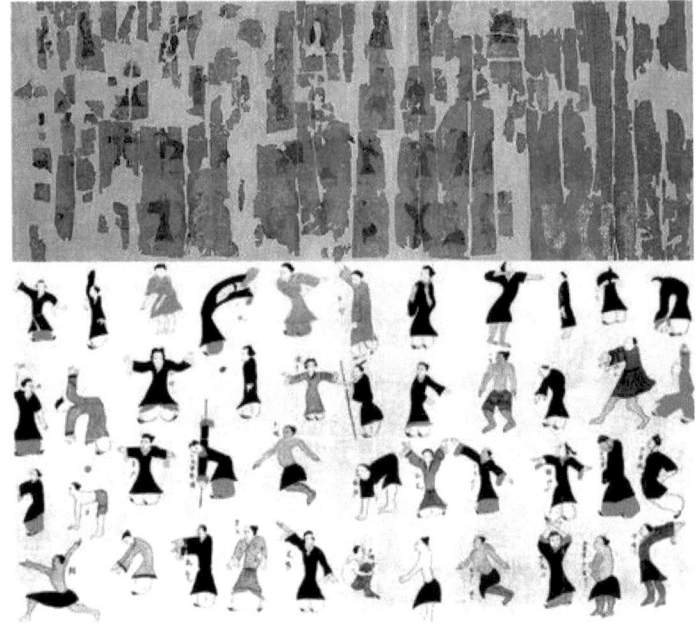

Figure 2

Figure 2 shows a silk image found in Changsha (China) in 1973. The site of discovery was the Han Dynasty Mawangdui Tomb, that was dated to 168 BC. The picture is called "Daoyintu" – "Instructions for exercises for guiding the Qi" and shows 44 people practicing various Qi Gong exercises.

How does Qi Gong affect the body?

Practicing Qi Gong improves self-awareness, balance, mobility and mindfulness with regard to everyday thinking and acting. This in turn leads to an improvement in body awareness and helps to achieve your individual feel-good weight.

A few years ago, researchers at the University of Queensland in Australia led by the physician Liu Xin carried out a study in which they had overweight people do Qi Gong exercises for three months. The result was that the test persons' blood pressure values improved and they significantly lost weight and waist circumference. And this without an additional strict diet or physical exertion.

Some explanations for this are as follows:

-The spiral movement sequences, which characterize the external exercises of Qi Gong, stimulate the muscles in a special way, so that more sugar is burned.
-The essence of Qi Gong is that an increased flow of Qi is stimulated throughout the body. This in turn leads to the fact that unneeded carbohydrates and fat reserves are used up.
-The body and its functions are brought into balance through Qi Gong. This allows the organs to do their work optimally, which is particularly helpful for people who suffer from a disorder here.
-By improving mindfulness, self-awareness and body awareness, people are able to listen better to their body – their "inner voice" – and to recognize what is healthy for them. As a result, behavioral changes are encouraged.

It is important to realize that all recognized Qi Gong exercises – i.e. also those while standing, sitting or lying down – are suitable for achieving health and a personal feel-good weight.

The Organ clock

The success of Qi Gong is based to a large extent on observation, perception, intuition and the resulting adaptation of the methods to one's own individual needs. Nevertheless, it is helpful to have a basic knowledge of theoretical foundations and facts.

In Traditional Chinese Medicine, it is assumed that the metabolic processes are subject to constant, cyclic change. This corresponds to the Daoist philosophy of the 5 phases of change (elements) wood, fire, earth, metal and water. This natural biological rhythm is represented by the so-called *Organ clock*. Accordingly, each organ has a period of maximum and minimum activity within the 24 hours of the day. If people observe the principles that can be derived from them, they are doing their body a favor and living in harmony with nature. If his lifestyle deviates significantly from this, this means stress for the organism, which can manifest itself in symptoms such as sleep disorders, tension, cardiovascular problems, lack of performance, lack of concentration and tiredness.

Figure 3 represents the TCM Organ clock. The individual time periods, functions and needs of the organs are outlined below.

1.Lungs
The lungs reach their greatest strength between 3 a.m. and 5 a.m. Traditionally, this period is considered the beginning of the daily cycle of the Organ clock. This is the time when the sleep hormone melotonin is released. Towards the end of the period, activity and dynamism slowly return to the body and blood pressure rises again.

The organ, on the other hand, reaches its lowest point between 3 p.m. and 5 p.m.

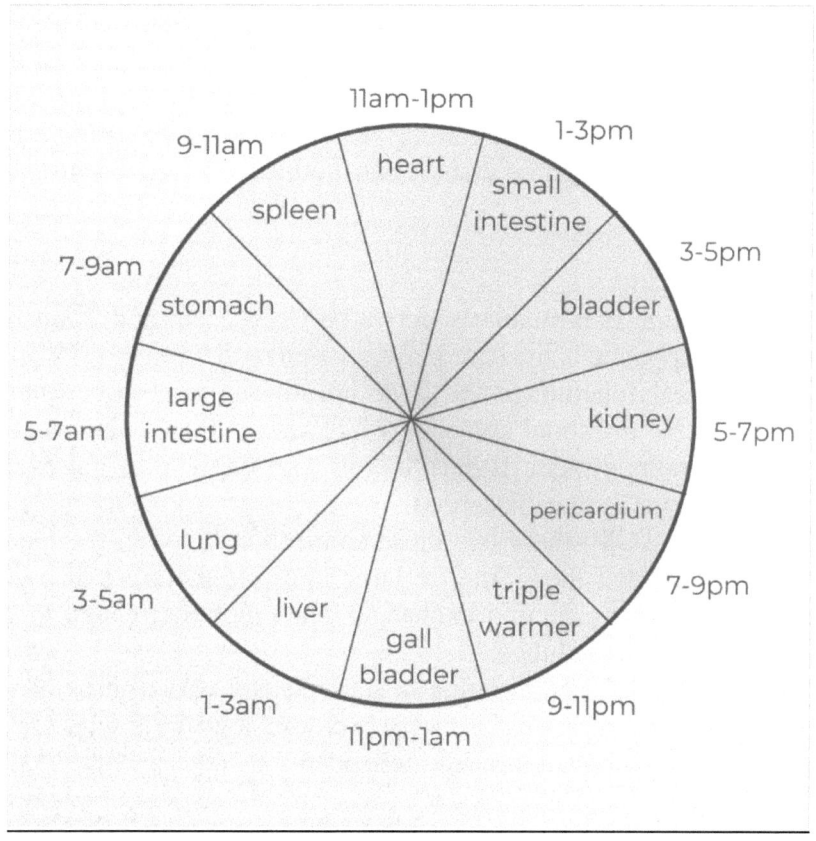

Figure 3

The lungs have the task of absorbing oxygen and then excreting carbon dioxide. Accordingly, it stands for absorbing as well as for letting go. The emotions of sadness, grief and melancholy are also associated with the lungs. It also stands for distance, courage and change.

With the breath, Qi is also absorbed into the body, which is why breathing is of great importance in Qi Gong. With their help, hunger and other feelings can also be regulated.

A good prophylaxis for the lungs is exercise in the fresh air (ideally in the mountains or by the sea, since the proximity of sand and stones is beneficial), laughing, sufficient sleep, break times, reducing stress and Qi Gong exercises that involve breathing. Recommended foods are e.g. hot ingredients and spices, game dishes, oat products, radishes, Harz cheese and peppermint tea.

2.The large intestine
The large intestine is particularly active between 5 am and 7 am in the morning. The opposite is the case between 5 pm and 7 pm.

The biological function of the large intestine is to absorb water and minerals from the intestinal contents, which means that it plays a central role in the immune system. It does its job with the help of gut bacteria. What is not needed is then discarded.

According to TCM, there is a close connection between the large in-testine, the lungs and the skin. The large intestine therefore also stands for acceptance, letting go and exchange. The emotions related to it are the same as those of the lungs.

It is good for the large intestine to start the day with a glass of warm water. In addition, exercise, Qi Gong exercises and the intake of foods suitable for the metabolism are recommended.

3.Stomach
The stomach is at its peak between 7 am and 9 am and at rest between 7 pm and 9 pm.

The stomach initially absorbs the food supplied to it in an uncon-trolled manner, whereby it can only feel very coarse stimuli. They are then broken up with the help of stomach acid, sterilized and finally passed on to the small intestine. The gastric mucosa protects its own cells from potentially harmful influences.

When the stomach is particularly active, digestion is in full swing, which is why we recommend taking a meal rich in carbohydrates. If you skip these despite feeling hungry, the organism reacts by reducing the metabolism and storing more energy reserves in the form of fat. The old saying applies here: "Breakfast like an emperor, lunch like a king, and dine like a beggar".

The stomach is emotionally associated with melancholy, brooding, hanging on to the past, as well as joie de vivre and greed. Hectic, suppressed anger, rage and dissatisfaction have a negative effect. The consumption of too much coffee, light wheat bread and sweets can also put a strain on the organ. On the other hand, calmness and patience, a balanced mind, regular meals that are not too late and generally a regular and orderly lifestyle have a positive influence.

4.Spleen-Pancreas

The spleen and pancreas are most active between 9 a.m. and 11 a.m. During this time the organism is very resistant. The rest of the two organs is between 9 p.m. and 11 p.m.

The spleen protects the inside of our body and acts as a bulwark against foreign objects. It also controls the red blood cells and breaks down older or unstable ones if necessary. The pancreas produces digestive juices and regulates blood sugar levels.

The organs represent the middle of the body and stand for a clear demarcation from the outside world and, conversely, for the development of one's own personality. In this sense, impulses and impressions are taken up and then transformed and further developed. Thoughtfulness and self-reflection are typical equivalents, as is the ability to interact socially with other people.

Worry is a burden. Food that is too cold, too fat and too carbohydrate-rich is also unfavorable, as is eating meals too late or too quickly.

The spleen is cared for through a balanced diet, exercise and relaxation, social contacts and gaining prestige, praise and recognition.

5.Heart

The heart peaks between 11 a.m. and 1 p.m. In this time window, it is advisable not to demand maximum performance from the body and to avoid great stress. Between 11 p.m. and 1 a.m. the organ is comparatively passive.

The heart is also known as the body's powerhouse because it pumps blood to all areas of the body. It has such a strong activity that it emits electromagnetic waves that energetically affect the environment. This corresponds to the scientific knowledge that the heart has its own nervous system and can make decisions independently of the brain.

In Far Eastern philosophy, however, it has another meaning: it is the seat of mind and soul and connects mind and body. It also stands for heat and fire in TCM.

The heart is very sensitive to negative feelings. This increases the stress hormone cortisol in the blood. This can go so far that diseases develop, brain cells are damaged, bone density decreases and fat is stored more quickly. Hectic, fast and excessive talking and sweating can also weaken the heart's energy.

Positive emotions, such as love, appreciation and sympathy, have a positive effect on the organ. This improves the heart rate and reduces the release of stress hormones. Corresponding emotions are joy, lust and love. Walks, phases of rest and, if necessary, well-seasoned food are also beneficial.

6. Small intestine

The small intestine is most active between 1 p.m. and 3 p.m. The so-called "midday slump" occurs during this time, as the blood is needed for digestion. Drugs can then have a prolonged effect, and rest or moderate exercise is more beneficial than exertion and exercise. The least activity of the organ takes place between 1 a.m. and 3 a.m.

In the small intestine, the ingested food is processed with the help of intestinal bacteria after it has remained in the stomach. This means that it is broken down into fats, proteins and sugar and a decision is made as to whether the components should be absorbed into the body or excreted. The individual cells that make up the intestine are tightly connected to prevent harmful substances from passing through and entering the organism.

Accordingly, the organ stands for careful analysis, the recognition of diversity and the courage to make decisions.

The small intestine can be affected by an intolerance to gluten, which puts a strain on the immune system, high amounts of fructose and abuse of painkillers or antibiotics. On the other hand, damaged intestinal wall cells can be rebuilt, e.g. through the intelligent administration of enzymes, zinc, vitamin C and L-glutamine.

Eating regular, not too large meals that are adapted to the metabolism is ideal for the intestines.

7. The bladder

The bladder works most intensively between 3 p.m. and 5 p.m. In this time window, the organism has a lot of power, oxygen and CO_2 available, so that the general performance is increased. Both physical and creative activities are therefore ideally possible. The organ has its lowest activity between 3 a.m. and 5 a.m.

The urinary bladder is the kidney's sister organ. It stands for self-orientation, stability and security. Since it serves to excrete fluid, it is necessary to drink enough.

8.The kidneys

The kidneys are at their peak activity between 5 p.m. and 7 p.m. Performance gradually decreases as the activity of the nerves that control the muscles decreases. The organ has its lowest point between 5 and 7 o'clock.

The kidney sucks fluid out of the body. Their task is to filter out harmful substances and, in cooperation with the bladder, to excrete them. There is therefore a connection between the kidneys, bladder, lungs, paranasal sinuses and the bone system. Admission and elimination as well as assessment and decision-making are typical features of the organ. For these reasons, the kidney is essential for the survival of the organism.

Her emotion is fear, which is a warning factor. In addition, it stands for willpower.

Severe heat and cold can impair the work of the kidneys, or the sensation of the same can be an indication of poor kidney function. Significant exertion and stress can also have a debilitating effect.

Rest and relaxation are good for the kidneys. In addition, she needs a sufficient amount of water every day in order to be able to do her job optimally.

9.Pericardium

The pericardium is particularly active between 7 p.m. and 9 p.m. The flow of blood is very strong during this time because it distributes the individual food components in the body. If the body is supplied with too many calories at the same time through food intake, then these are stored very quickly as fat tissue, since the stomach has its rest period. The main organs of the body therefore need rest and recovery. The period of time in which the organ is comparatively passive is between 7 a.m. and 9 a.m.

The pericardium has the task of protecting the heart and regulating its expansion.

The pericardium is supported in its work by the supply of fresh oxygen, e.g. during a walk, on the terrace or at the window.

18

10.Triple burner

The triple burner has its peak time between 9 pm and 11 pm. During this period, the body is most relaxed. At the same time, the immune system is particularly active. The period of rest is from 9 a.m. to 11 a.m.

The so-called "Triple burner" is a meridian that has no anatomical, organic equivalent. It is an energy pathway that is responsible for the heat regulation of the entire body.

The meridian stands for the harmony between the inside and the outside, for the balance between dreams, wishes and thoughts on the one hand and activity in the here and now on the other.

The cells regenerate during the time when the Triple burner reaches its highest level of activity. It is therefore recommended not to eat or drink anything and to avoid any stress on the organism.

11.The gallbladder

The gallbladder is at its peak between 11 p.m. and 1 a.m. and is at its lowest between 11 a.m. and 1 p.m.

The gallbladder forms a functional unit together with the liver. It detoxifies the body and helps with fat digestion and constipation. Accordingly, it stands for decision-making power and determination.

Emotions attributed to the gallbladder are anger, rage, depression and irritation. In addition, it corresponds to an aggression that serves self-preservation, the removal of obstacles and further development. Consequently, it can create good confidence and self-esteem.

During periods of increased gallbladder activity, the body primarily needs rest and time to regenerate itself. If, on the other hand, he is still exposed to a lot of stimuli, exertion or food and drink that is difficult to digest, this can lead to after-pains the following day, such as a lack of alertness and presence.

12.Liver

The liver is at its peak between 1a.m. and 3 a.m. Traditionally, this period is considered the conclusion of the daily cycle of the Organ clock. The organ's rest period is between 3 p.m. and 5 p.m.

The liver is the largest metabolic organ. On the one hand, it produces vital vitamins, proteins and minerals and passes them on to other parts of the body. On the other hand, it protects the internal organs and the bloodstream from substances that put a strain on the organism by excreting them in the bile. It is therefore associated with transformation, change and renewal. According to the holistic way of thinking of TCM, this applies both organically and spiritually.

It is said that the liver regulates emotions and feelings in general. Typical emotions and characteristics that correspond to it are anger, resentment, bitterness, the adaptability of one's ideas and values and the ability to draw boundaries and define one's own living space. Liver weakness can lead to fatigue and exhaustion. But muscle, tendon and joint diseases can also be associated with it.

The liver is stressed by eating late, high-calorie meals, drinking too much alcohol or not getting enough sleep. Too many cold foods and drinks can also have an unfavorable effect.

The period of the highest activity of the liver means the lowest point of physical performance. One should give the body rest for self-cleansing and detoxification. In general, the careful choice of digestible foods is recommended.

What can we learn from the Organ clock?

According to Traditional Chinese Medicine, the Organ clock ticks equally for everyone. The corresponding metabolic processes have developed in the course of evolution over many thousands of years and are therefore of general validity. It is therefore of great advantage to have at least a basic understanding of the cyclical processes within the body, which involve periods of activity and periods of rest.

Nevertheless, the properties listed above and the resulting recommendations for action are only to be understood as points of reference and guidelines and not as irrefutable dogmas. In our time it is only possible for very few people to strictly adhere to the rules of nutrition, health exercises and rhythm of life. The demands of work and everyday life are too enormous, too diverse and too varied for that. Everything in life is constantly in flux, so adjustments and the art of improvisation are always needed. For example, if you get up later, you naturally cannot have breakfast at 8 a.m. Anyone who comes to dinner late in the evening due to all-day commitments can only do so to a limited extent and must comply with the times available to them. If you work in shifts or travel a lot, you sometimes have to adjust your nutrition plan every day.

The mere knowledge of the existence of the Organ clock and of certain needs of our organs and their functional circuits is at least a beginning. Moreover, to a certain extent, our body is quite capable of getting used to the respective living conditions, i.e. to compensate for deviations from the ideal state. In addition, we have other tools at our disposal to increase our physical well-being, such as Qi Gong and Dietetics.

Dietetics

Dietetics is the part of traditional Chinese medicine that deals with nutritional therapy. Food intake is therefore considered from the point of view that it serves to prevent and treat diseases. Here, too, the holistic approach applies that physical and mental aspects must be in harmony with each other. Furthermore, it is considered a fact that the life energy Qi is absorbed through food. Strictly speaking, Qi is formed from food and then mixed with air and distributed throughout the body.

Dietetics should not be confused with the characteristics of a diet in the traditional sense. Most diets that are created according to the findings of Western medicine primarily rely on the following three properties: renunciation (of calories) + time component (quick goal achievement and time limit) + weight reduction as the primary or only goal. Unfortunately, this form of controlling food intake rarely has the desired long-term effect (keyword "yo-yo effect") and also has some health risks.

Qi Gong, TCM and Dietetics have always taken a different path. They begin by acknowledging the fact that every human being is an individual with very specific, unique nutritional needs. Furthermore, the way we eat, with the help of which our body gains important energy resources, should be designed in such a way that we are able to maintain it permanently and not just for a short time. Visible successes can therefore sometimes only appear after a while, but are lasting and constant. And finally, food intake, lifestyle, energetic exercises, etc. should always be considered under the higher goal of health, i.e. losing weight should not be an end in itself, but should serve to improve performance, well-being and inner functional cycles.

If the person is basically healthy, then it is not necessary to take additional medication, dietary supplements, etc. It is always better when our body and mind achieve health and healing through their own initiative and strength.

In "Huangdi Neijing Suwen", the "Yellow Emperor's Classic on Internal Medicine" by Huang Di it says:

"One should only ever partially heal diseases with the help of drugs with medicinal properties. The completion of healing is attained by eating the grains, meats and vegetables. In this way, damage to the vital force is avoided and the risk of overdoses and side effects is reduced."

General rules of nutrition

One of the basic rules of nutrition according to TCM and the principles of Qi Gong is to identify those foods and diets that are favorable for one's own metabolism. The most important tools for this are intuition and self-awareness, i.e. the ability to recognize the needs of our body. In addition, of course, there are some facts that are part of generally accepted knowledge.

With regard to our physical well-being and achieving a feel-good weight, it goes without saying that the consumption of carbohydrates and fats must be in reasonable proportion to the calorie consumption. Except for rare cases, anyone who constantly consumes excess calories will find it difficult not to increase or even reduce their body weight. The reverse case basically leads to a reduction in physical mass. However, the question arises as to whether abstinence can be seen as positive for physical and mental health and whether such a diet can be sustained in the long term or only has a temporary effect.

Furthermore, with diets that rely on forgoing food intake, it is often forgotten that this can lead to a slowdown in metabolism and increased storage of fatty tissue. Since the body knows that it is getting little energy, it stores it as fat as an emergency reserve.

The food you eat should be of high quality and fresh. Good carbohydrates are complex in nature and can be found, for example, in whole grain products, potatoes or brown rice. Due to their molecular structure, the body needs more time to break them down and obtain energy from them, so that the blood sugar level remains constant. Sources of valuable proteins are lean meat and fish as well as legumes such as beans and lentils, seeds and nuts. Healthy fats are those that are high in omega 3 or oleic acids. Suppliers for this are e.g. walnuts, linseed, cheese, salmon, eggs, olive and rapeseed oil, yoghurt and dark chocolate. Fresh fruit and vegetables should be selected according to seasonal and regional aspects.

Warm foods, e.g. steamed vegetables, are easier for the body to digest and require less energy than cold foods, e.g. those from the refrigerator or raw vegetables. In general, therefore, warm, briefly cooked dishes with little fat are recommended. This can include grains and vegetables, as well as smaller amounts of oils, meat, fish and dairy products.

As far as the amount of food consumed or the size of the food is concerned, the needs of people vary greatly. Eating too little causes a lack of energy reserves, the shutting down of the metabolism and psychological stress. Eating too much food overloads the pancreas and leads to the storage of fat reserves. Here you should follow a simple rule: Eat when and as long as you are hungry!

Anyone who refuses to eat despite feeling hungry is acting against their nature and is doing their body and mind no good. On the other hand, you should not overdo it, e.g. for reasons of enjoyment, and regularly "fill your stomach". In Qi Gong one speaks of the 70% rule. This means that you should only ever strain yourself up to this limit and not up to the maximum capacity. You should also take this to heart when eating. If you find that you have almost reached the state of saturation, then you should stop and do without another second helping, which would inevitably put a strain on the organism. The people living in the Okinawa region of Japan, known for their long life expectancy, have always adhered to this principle.

With regard to the ideal meal times, it is possible to use the Organ clock as a guide. As we have seen above, our body can best utilize food between 7 and 9 a.m., while in the evening it prefers smaller portions or lighter food and at night rest and abstinence are needed (between 1 a.m. and 3 a.m. is the peak of the liver). On the other hand, however, it is important to adapt the times of food intake to your own daily routine. An important indication that your stomach is working properly is that you feel hungry at constant intervals or at the same time of day. When the stomach sends signals of hunger, it is ready to receive food. This should be heeded and not ignored.

In any case, you should make sure that you allow yourself enough time and rest to eat and have fun with it. Taking meals correctly means sitting down, blocking out disturbing and stressful thoughts and concentrating entirely on eating. Chew thoroughly and enjoy mindfully and consciously. On the other hand, you should avoid strenuous discussions or arguments with your neighbors at the table and instead try to treat your family or friends with love and respect.

Another essential piece of advice is: observe how you feel after you eat!

If you're feeling good about the type, amount, and timing of your meals, then you're most likely already doing something right. If you regularly experience bloating, leaden heaviness, nausea, etc. perceive, then you should consider changes here or there. In this regard, they should be attentive and honest with themselves.

There is a saying that after a meal one should rest or go for a walk. I have to agree. When the organism is engaged in digestion, it should be kept away from exertion and stress for a while. Moderate exercise supports the metabolism, but relaxation is also essential. Physical as well as mental strength are not inexhaustible, and a deficiency can lead to immune deficiencies, sleep disorders, anxiety, concentration problems and a loss of inner balance.

Still water, tap water or herbal tea are recommended for drinking. The kidneys need enough fluid to eliminate unneeded substances from the body. However, it is difficult to set a minimum quantity. Drinking warm water saves energy that the stomach would otherwise need to heat the liquid to a usable temperature.

You should not drink too much immediately before or while eating, as this affects the feeling of satiety and the stomach is fooled into thinking that it is getting usable food. Although this leads to a suppression of the feeling of hunger, it also leads to an energy deficit. In the sense of TCM and Qi Gong, acting against nature is never to be seen as sensible.

Classification of food

According to Dietetics, there are no foods that are fundamentally good or bad. Instead, the effect is considered, which can be moderate or quite extreme. A balanced composition of the ingredients of a meal is aimed for in the following. Here, too, a holistic approach applies - as is usual in all areas of TCM.

The two most important differentiation criteria are the classifications into cold and hot (thermal effect) and into wet and dry (see Figure 4).

cold	hot
wet	dry

Figure 4

Cold foods include, for example, green tea, cucumbers, zucchini, yoghurt, ice cream, pears, salt, mineral water, beer, tomatoes, soy sauce, asparagus, zucchini, pumpkin, saffron, sorrel, crab, algae, watermelon, paprika, lemon, quark, banana, endive, tofu and venison.

Herbal tea, apples, wheat, broccoli, lettuce, blackberries, soybeans, tofu, duck, turkey, goose, sauerkraut, cauliflower, mango, orange, sunflower oil, jam, pork, cress, plums, corn, kohlrabi, legumes, peppermint and celery are not quite as cold (cool).

Spinach, millet, asparagus, rye, green beans, radishes, sweet potatoes, plaice, mushrooms, lamb's lettuce, aubergines, tangerines, peas, cheese, avocado, sugar, raspberries, oats, Brussels sprouts, butter, Safflower oil, cooked grains, bread, pasta, rice, eggs, sour milk products, potatoes, carrots, mushrooms, grapes, figs, nuts, beef and black tea have a neutral effect.

Not too hot (warm) are, for example, cocoa, milk, wine, coconut milk, vinegar, beetroot, leeks, onions, dried herbs and spices, sunflower seeds, peaches, papaya, plums, strawberries, cherries, fish, chicken, pumpkin, . raisins, apricots, garlic, dill and ginger.

Hot foods are strong alcoholic drinks, fennel, white radish, chili, pineapple, hot spices, grilled meat, pepper, nutmeg, spiced teas, coffee, cinnamon, thyme, anise, goat's/sheep's cheese, bitter chocolate, sausage, cloves, vinegar, curry and cardamom.

The thermal effect of a food always remains the same. This means that a cucumber is always cold, regardless of whether it is eaten warm or cold, and a chili pepper stays hot, regardless of the temperature at which it is served.

Wet foods include fatty and sweet foodstuff, as well as dairy and raw foods. Examples are sweet alcohol, cow's milk cheese, chocolate, nuts, honey, dates, oils, avocados, jam, quark, banana, yoghurt, beer, raspberries, mineral water, pears, tofu, melon, watercress, pork, goose, duck, apples, mangoes, oranges, sauerkraut, spinach, tangerines, peas, butter, Brussels sprouts, milk, grapes, raisins, figs, apricots and fish and sausages with a high fat content.

Thyme, rosemary, basil, ginger, tabasco, oregano, celery, rye, coffee, strong alcoholic drinks, nutmeg, spiced teas, pepper, grilled meat, crab, seaweed, green and black tea, some types of mushrooms, peppermint, asparagus, green beans, oats, wheat, fennel, parsley, dill, leeks, coriander, cardamom, cinnamon and cloves as well as hot and spicy foods in general are considered dry.

Sheep and goat meat and cheese, lean sausage, dry wine, curry, low-fat fish, peppers, garlic, chestnuts, cherries, peaches, carrots, beef, shrimp, chicken, strawberries, pumpkin, rice, pasta, bread, lamb's lettuce, white mushrooms, eggplant, broccoli, tomatoes, lemons, zucchini, sorrel, cucumbers, melons, cabbages, blackberries, lemons, potatoes, radishes, legumes and corn are neutral in this regard.

The goal when putting together the meals should be that they are balanced with regard to the above classifications. This is the case when most of the food is in the respective neutral area. If possible, you should avoid using only extremely rated foods, because this leads to one-sidedness or an arc of tension and can bring the body into imbalance. This in turn can have a wide range of unfavorable consequences in the long term, such as lack of energy and performance, tiredness, forgetfulness, irritability, headaches, an increase in blood pressure, blood fat and blood sugar and of course obesity with all the associated side effects

It is not necessary for you to memorize the classification of all the above foods. It should be enough if you are aware of the effects of the ones you use most often. In addition, with mindfulness and a little experience, in many cases you can tell for yourself whether something you are eating feels hot or cold, wet or dry. It is important that you develop the right awareness of the topic and always observe how you feel after meals. Over time, this will undoubtedly help you to eat more consciously, more balanced and healthier.

According to the Daoist philosophy, all things and processes in the universe can be described using *5 elements* or *5 elementary phases of change*. These 5 elements are

1. Wood
2. Fire
3. Earth
4. Metal
5. Water.

According to this model, each of the elements is assigned a specific flavor (see Figure 5). It refers to

1. sour
2. bitter
3. sweet
4. pungent
5. salty

FIVE ELEMENT THEORY

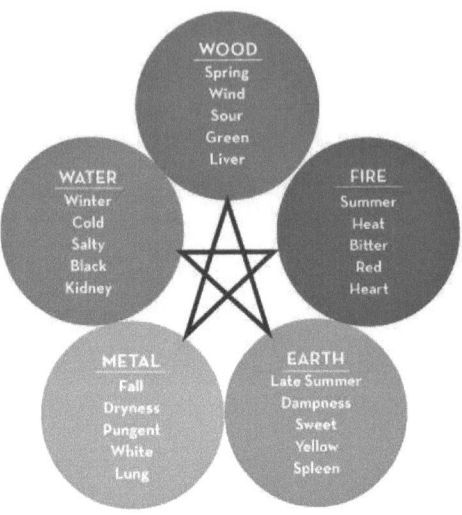

Figure 5

Acidic foods have a preservative and calming effect on the body, causing growth and providing flexibility. Examples are lemons, oranges and apples.

Bitter foods have a draining, detoxifying and anti-inflammatory effect. Examples are coffee, tea, chard, spinach, artichokes, ginger, olives, eggplant, some herbs such as dandelion and nettle, and spices such as turmeric, mustard seeds, thyme and cinnamon.

Sweet foods provide general energy and have a relaxing effect. Examples are sugar, sweet fruits and cooked grains.

Pungent foods stimulate movement in the body, dissolve blockages, have a drying effect and are used to cleanse (e.g. the lungs). Examples are chillies, horseradish, leeks and mustard.

Salty foods are expectorant, provide cleansing and aid in digestion. Examples are salt, shellfish and some vegetables, such as celery.

If you eat from all five flavors, then the body is in balance and can work optimally. This doesn't mean that you have to fit all of the flavors into a single meal, but that you should alternate and vary this from time to time. In Chinese cuisine, for example, two variants are often combined with each other, such as sweet and sour or salty and pungent, etc. Furthermore, the suppliers of the above flavors are to be regarded as extremes, i.e. they should not dominate the entire meal, but always form only one nuance. Too much salt is known to be bad for blood pressure, too much sugar is bad for blood sugar and teeth, and not everyone can tolerate a lot of spiciness. Just make sure that they offer the palate a different taste experience from time to time, then you have a good chance of satisfying the 5-element model of TCM and keeping the inner processes in your body in balance and momentum.

Dishes based on Dietetics

Typical ingredients that are used in Chinese cuisine and correspond to the principles of Dietetics or TCM are the following:

-Garlic: purifies the blood, promotes digestion
-Ginger: strengthen the kidneys -Wheat germ oil, soybean oil: cell regenerating
-Onions, shallots: antibacterial, antibiotic
-Rice wine: strengthens the cardiovascular system.

In addition, the following medicinal plants, herbs and fruits are recommended for regular consumption:

Thermal effect cold:
-Aloe Vera
-Bananas
-Chrysanthemum
-Cucumbers
-Dandelion
-Peppermint
-Black sesame
-Watermelon.

Thermal effect warm:
-Angelica Root
-Fennel
-Dates
-Rosemary
-Walnut
-Nutmeg
-Coriander
-Ginseng.

Then you will find some dishes that can be prepared with relatively moderate effort. They are balanced according to the standards of Chinese Dietetics and are therefore suitable for incorporation into your diet plan. The recipes are only exemplary in nature and should serve as inspiration. You can of course modify them according to your preference, taste and availability of the ingredients. The cooking times differ depending on the quantity and size of the ingredients, temperature, etc. Furthermore, the dishes can be supplemented with a side dish, e.g. rice or salad.

Ginger chicken with rice wine

-Ingredients: Butter or Oil, Ginger, Chicken Leg (or other chicken parts), Corn, Paprika Powder, Curry, Pepper, Salt, Rice Wine

-Preparation: Heat butter/oil in a pan, briefly sauté the chopped ginger over low heat; Add the chicken leg, sprinkle with paprika powder and fry on all sides; Pour rice wine and add corn; sprinkle all with curry powder and simmer for a few minutes until the meat is cooked; season with salt and pepper

Leek pan with tofu

-Ingredients: 1 celeriac, leeks, carrots, oil, vegetable broth, onions, potatoes, tofu, paprika powder, pepper, salt

-Preparation: Chop the leeks and onions, dice the celery, potatoes and tofu; heat oil in a pan, sprinkle the tofu with paprika powder and sauté for about 20 minutes; heat about 250 ml vegetable stock in a saucepan and cook the potatoes, celery, onions, carrots and leeks for about 20 minutes until the carrots are soft; add the tofu cubes and season with salt and pepper

Meat with sweet and sour sauce

-Ingredients: beef or pork, ginger, onion, beans, soybean oil, rice wine, chicken or vegetable broth, flour, sugar, vinegar, salt, pepper

-Preparation: cut the meat into thin strips and roll in flour; Mix chopped ginger, chopped onions, some broth, rice wine, vinegar and sugar in a bowl; Sear the meat in a pan in soybean oil, add the beans and then let it stew for a few minutes; Stir in the sauce and let it thicken a bit

Chicken soup

-Ingredients: 1 soup chicken, bunch of soup greens, ginger, chives, garlic cloves, 250 – 300 g rice, salt

-Preparation: cook the chicken, greens, chopped garlic and ginger in about 2 liters of salted water for about 1 1/2 hours over a low heat; sieve the broth and skim off the fat; add the boiled rice, season with chopped parsley; if desired, the meat can be removed from the bone and returned to the soup

Fish with paprika mushroom vegetables

-Ingredients: 500 g redfish fillet (alternatively pollock or cod), red peppers, mushrooms, shallots or onions, clove of garlic, chicken or vegetable stock, vinegar, rice wine, soy sauce, tomato paste, 1 pinch each of salt, pepper and sugar

-Preparation: soak dried fish fillets in rice wine for a few minutes; heat the oil in a pan and sauté the garlic and onions, add the fish and stew for about 20 minutes; cut the peppers and mushrooms into strips and fry them in a pan; mix some broth, tomato paste, soy sauce and vinegar and pour over the vegetables; finally pour the paprika and mushroom sauce over the fish

Vegetable turkey curry with coconut milk

-Ingredients: 50 - 100 g fragrant or sticky rice, 100 ml chicken stock, 100 ml coconut milk, turkey escalope or tofu, oil, mushrooms, peas, onion, coriander, salt, pepper, flour, curry powder

-Preparation: heat oil in a pan and fry diced meat or tofu in it, salt and pepper; fry mushrooms and onions in a pan, dust with flour and curry and pour in coconut milk and broth; add the peas and cook over a low heat for a few minutes; season with coriander, salt and pepper; add the coconut milk sauce to the meat and let it simmer

Chili sine carne
-Ingredients: canned corn, kidney beans, canned tomatoes or beefsteak tomatoes and tomato paste, red and green peppers, 1 chili pepper, garlic, onion, sugar, turmeric, paprika powder, salt, pepper
-Preparation: heat some oil in a pan and fry the diced onions, paprika, chili and garlic; add the beans and tomatoes and simmer until the beans are cooked; season with paprika powder, turmeric, sugar, salt and pepper

Falafel
-Ingredients: approx. 300 g chickpeas (from the tin or leave to soak for approx. 24 hours beforehand), onions, garlic cloves, 1 chili, turmeric, 1 bunch of parsley, cumin
-Preparation: Finely chop the onions, garlic, chili and chickpeas and pu-ree in a blender or with an immersion blender; season with cumin, salt and turmeric and fold in the chopped parsley; knead small balls from the mixture and fry or deep-fry in hot oil; any dip goes well with it

Healthy herbal teas

In addition to water, herbal teas are most suitable for covering the liquid requirement. They also have the advantage that their valuable ingredients such as vitamins, minerals and enzymes can have a positive effect on our health. The following varieties are particularly recommended in China and according to TCM standards.

Green tea
Green tea is generally considered to be the healthiest drink (see Figure 6). It owes its stimulating effect to caffeine.
-Brewing time: 1-2 min.
-Effect: vitamins, improvement of blood pressure, blood fat, cholesterol and blood sugar levels, lowering the risk of heart attack

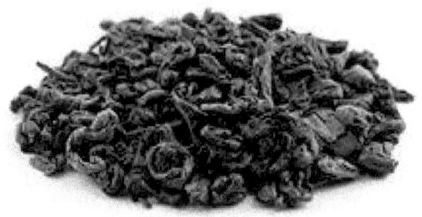

Figure 6

Pu-erh tea

The red Pu-Erh tea is considered to be the oldest type of tea in human history.
-Steeping time: approx. 1 min.; the leaves can be boiled several times
-Effect: favorably influences metabolism, detoxifies, purifies, stimulates digestion, strengthens the immune system, has a favorable influence on nutrition-related diseases

Jiaogulan tea
In the region where Jiaogulan grows, people are considered to be particularly long-lived, which is why it is also known as the "immortality herb".
-Steeping time: approx. 10 minutes; a small amount of the herbs will suffice
-Effect: has a calming effect on stress, difficulty falling asleep and high blood pressure, lowers blood sugar levels and blood lipid levels, has a haematopoietic effect, may have an anti-cancer effect and strengthens the immune system

Oolong tea
Ooolong tea is also considered a slimming aid, as studies have shown that its consumption improves metabolism and increases energy metabolism.

36

-Steeping time: approx. 3 min.; with another infusion you can extend the brewing time
-Effect: increase in energy metabolism, lowering of blood sugar levels, protection of blood vessels from dangerous deposits, strengthening of the immune system, antibacterial effect, prevents skin aging

Ginseng tea
Ginseng is considered one of the most nutrient dense foods in the world. It has been used in Chinese and Korean medicine for thousands of years. It should not be confused with the "Siberian ginseng" (taiga root).
-Steeping time: approx. 5-10 min.
-Effect: Strengthening of the immune system, antioxidant effect, increase in mental performance and concentration, reduction of stress symptoms

Ginger tea
Ginger has long been known in the western hemisphere as part of exotic foods such as Sushi. Ginger is not only used in Chinese cuisine, but also in TCM due to its positive health effects.
-Steeping time: approx. 5-10 min.
-Effect: supplier of vitamin C and many minerals, antibacterial and anti-inflammatory, stimulation of blood flow and circulation, promotion of digestion and metabolism

Nettle tea
The stinging nettle plant is widespread throughout the northern hemisphere. Although it is often misjudged as a weed, its high medicinal benefits are now undisputed.
-Steeping time: approx. 5 min.
-Effect: inhibits inflammation and bacteria, diuretic, draining, purifying, detoxifying, alleviates hay fever and other allergies, vitamin A and C, strengthens the immune system

Qi Gong exercises

The practical exercises presented below are all very well suited to maximizing the life energy we have and optimizing the flow of Qi in our body. In this way, the metabolic processes are boosted and superfluous energy is utilized. They are of an exemplary nature, i.e. you can, for example, choose further exercises from my book series "Stay young with Qi Gong!" and integrate them into your personal training program. In these volumes you will also find a lot of general information, e.g. on breathing, the preparatory Qi Gong state or the ideal framework for the practice session.

There are standing exercises ("The 8 Brocades while standing", "The 18 Tai Chi Exercises"), sitting ("The 8 Brocades while sitting", "The small Heavenly circuit", "The Embryo Breathing"), walking ("Daoist circle walking", "The Game of the 5 animals") as well as lying down ("Bone marrow Qi Gong"). These are all suitable to achieve your goals.

Regularity is an essential principle for the success of the exercise. Endurance and perseverance are just as important. If you have found some Qi Gong exercises that you like, then ideally set a fixed time of day when you can devote yourself to them undisturbed. Avoid over-ambition and only practice as long as you feel good and enjoy it. In Qi Gong one speaks of the "70% rule", which means that you should never go to the limit of your stress potential, as this would have an energetically counterproductive effect. Furthermore, you should not expose yourself to any time pressure, because Qi Gong is intended to be practiced continuously. The successes for health and physical well-being will therefore be all the more sustainable.

The stance with which almost every Qi Gong training begins is sometimes referred to as the "Wuji stance". Wuji is an important term in Daoist terminology and is translated as "peak of nothing" or "the infinite".

Place your feet parallel and shoulder-width apart. The imaginary line from the highest point of the shoulders (Jianjing acupuncture point) through the outside of the pelvis to the sole of the foot (Yongquan Qi Gong point) should be a vertical line. The feet are evenly loaded and give a feeling as if they were firmly rooted in the ground. The associated Qi Gong motto is: "Empty at the top, solid at the bottom". This means that in the upper part of the body there is lightness and emptiness, while the lower part (Lower Dantian, kwa, legs) ensures firmness and inner strength. The natural model is the structure and function of a tree.

After completing a Qi Gong exercise, the Qi is always collected in the Lower Dantian, which is located below the navel. To do this, place both palms on top of each other on this area for a while, with women placing the left hand on the right and men placing the right hand on the left. Alternatively, raise both hands in front of your chest while inhaling and slowly lower them while exhaling.

A Qi Gong motto is: "Imagination moves the Qi, and the Qi moves the blood." Thus, when you perform one of the above concluding exercises, the life energy is guided to its natural storage location, the Lower Dantian, where it can be called up when needed can be.

The Daoist Cloud hands

Since the 10th of the 18 Tai Chi exercises is also called "Cloud hands", we are talking about the "Daoist" Cloud hands to make it easier to differentiate between them.

After reaching the Qi Gong state, stand in a neutral position (Wuji stance). The footwork consists of first turning to your left side, whereby the weight is completely shifted to the left leg and the right leg is relieved. It is said that the loaded leg becomes "full" (with weight) and the other "empty". Then return to the center and move to the right. The feet remain firmly rooted in the ground. The same footwork is used for the first swing exercise.

When doing the twist, it is important that you do not initiate it with your shoulders or core muscles, but with what the Chinese call "Kwa". This includes the area of the pelvis including the internal organs and associated muscles as well as the inguinal ligaments. You should also make sure that the upper body always remains straight, i.e. the shoulders must be in a vertical line above the hips.

To perform the complete exercise, initially take both hands in front of your chest, with the palms facing each other (see Figure 7).

When turning the body to the left, the right hand now rises to the top left, while the left hand is brought straight down to the left hip. The palms always point in the direction of movement, and the gaze follows the rising hand. Inhale during this part of the exercise (see Figure 8).

As you exhale, turn your body back to the center, whereupon the movement is carried out smoothly to the other side on the subsequent inhalation. The sequence of movements is never stopped after the exercise has started, i.e. there is no lingering in the starting position. Consequently, over time, the practitioner needs to get a feel for the right timing and coordination of movement and breathing.

The Daoist Cloud hands have many positive effects and are considered a very comprehensive Qi Gong exercise. Through the shift in weight and the spiral movements, the various parts of our body experience an opening and closing, stretching and bending, screwing and turning. In addition, the body is energetically connected to the spine, the Qi flow is stimulated and the internal organs are massaged, so to speak. Due to the soft and slow character of the movements, our mind is relaxed and a lot of fresh Qi is absorbed. In Qi Gong, helical movements are moreover often described as "the spinning of the silk thread".

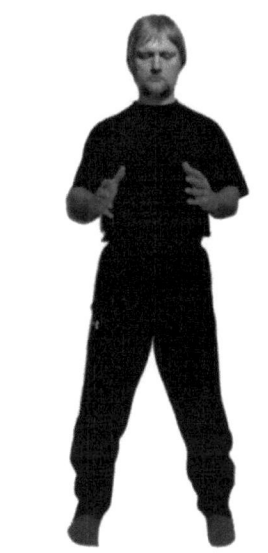

Figure 7

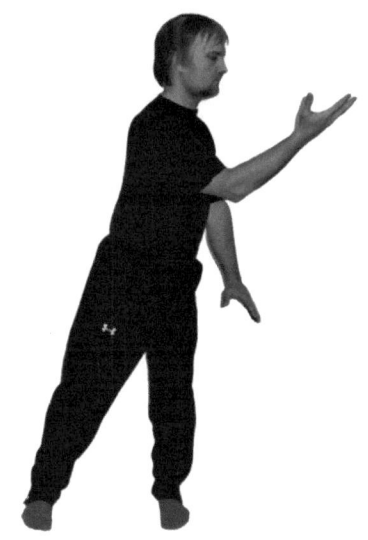

Figure 8

1st Brocade while standing: Hold up the sky

In the starting position, the hands form a shell in front of the lower abdomen, with the palms facing up and the fingertips at a slight distance from each other (see Figure 9).

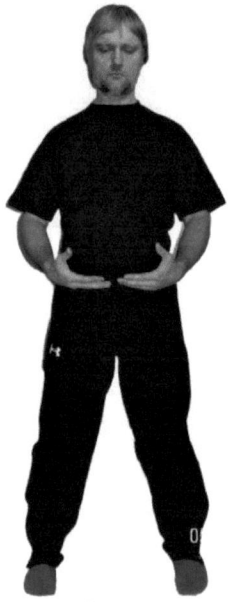

Figure 9

As you inhale, move your arms up in a straight line. The forearms turn once around their own axis from chest height so that the thumbs point forward and the little fingers are facing the body. Finally, your arms rise above your head in a loosely bent position. The arms and hands have now reached a supportive position, and the gaze also goes up to the sky. During this process, the body is lifted or stretched a little while the feet remain firmly on the ground (see Figure 10).

When you then exhale, the arms make a circular motion to the sides with the palms facing outwards. Eventually they return to their original position. During this process, the knees are bent again so that the body's center of gravity is lowered.

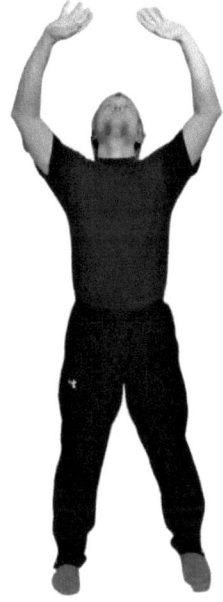

Figure 10

3rd Tai Chi exercise: Moving the Rainbow

The exercise begins in the normal Wuji stance. When inhaling for the first time, both arms are brought straight up in front of the body. Let your hands hang loosely. Finally, the arms protrude almost straight up, with the palms of the hands facing inwards. The view remains directed forward (see Figure 11).

As you exhale, all of your body weight is shifted to your right leg and your left hand is moved outward to about the level of your shoulders. The right hand is now over the top of the head so that both palms are still facing each other. The gaze is oriented towards the left hand. You can hold this position for a few moments (see Figure 12).

The next time you inhale, you return to the starting position. Then the movement is repeated to the other side.

If you like, you can imagine moving a rainbow between your hands as you perform the exercise. This ensures great inner peace.

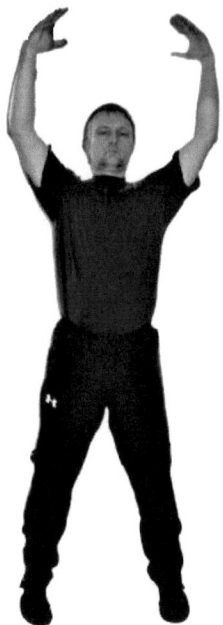

Figure 11

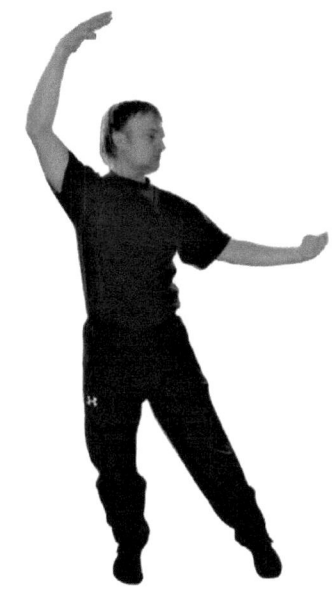

Figure 12

18th Tai Chi exercise: Filling Qi into the body

The last of the 18 Tai Chi exercises is also the ideal final exercise in the series, regardless of whether you have previously performed all or only selected individual exercises. It is also known under the name "Calming the Qi" and thus brings full circle, because the 1st exercise is called "Awakening the Qi".

Of course - as explained in volume 1 of the series - it can also serve as a final exercise for all possible Qi Gong practices. In addition, it represents one of the most beneficial and complete Qi Gong exercises of all. The three Qi Gong principles *movement + imagination + breathing* are perfectly synchronized with each other and ensure that fresh Qi is in the body down to the Lower Dantian is promoted and at the same time used up Qi is led outside.

When breathing in, both arms are brought from the starting position laterally in a large, circular movement over the head. The palms of the hands are facing upwards. Finally, the hands form a roof (see Figure 13).

When exhaling very slowly, both hands are brought vertically down in front of the body to the Lower Dantian. The gaze accompanies the movement (see Figure 14).

You can repeat this process as often as you like. Then switch to the second and final part of the exercise.

While breathing in, both hands are spread laterally in front of the body, as if you were hugging a large (Qi) ball.

During the subsequent exhalation, bring both hands towards the body until they finally come to rest on the lower abdomen. Women place their right hand first and the left hand over it, for men it is the other way round (see Figure 15).

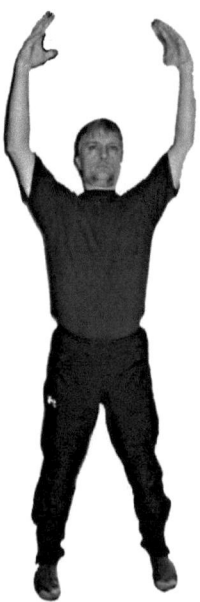

Figure 13

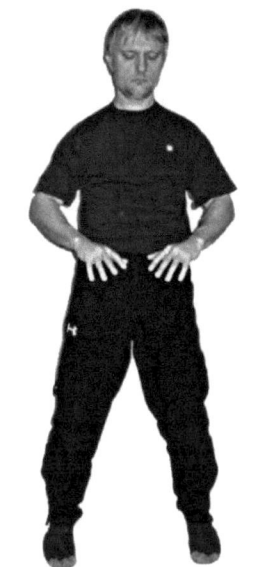

Figure 14

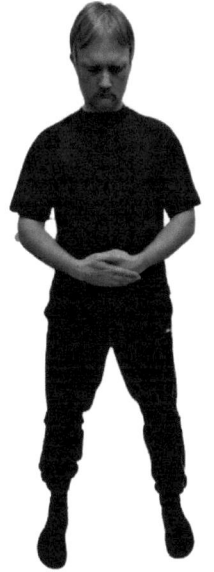

Figure 15

Close your eyes and keep your attention on the most important Qi Gong point, the Lower Dantian, for a while. Continue to breathe in your normal abdominal breathing.

During the first or the main part of the exercise, as you breathe in, you can imagine that your arms are reaching far out into the universe and scooping a large amount of fresh energy into the area above your head. The Qi compressed there is then filled into the body through the apex when exhaling, directed downwards and stored in the Lower Dantian. Through the soles of the feet (bubbling spring points), used up Qi is brought out at the same time.

2nd Preparatory exercise of the Lohan Qi Gong: Absorbing energy with your hands

From the Wuji stand, take your left hand a little behind your body and turn accordingly in this direction (Figure 16).

Then the hand is moved upwards and forwards with the palm facing upwards until it is roughly in front of the shoulder. The body axis will be straightened again (see Figure 17).

Now turn your palm down and move your left hand down and to the right until you reach your right hip. The body is also turned in this direction. At the same time, take your right hand a little behind your body.

Then repeat the sequence of movements to the other side by first moving your right hand up and then down to the left. You can then continue this process as you wish

The gaze follows the course of the moving hand.

This exercise is very effective and brings a lot of fresh energy into the body via the Lao Gung points on the palms of the hands. In addition, the torso and the extremities are energetically connected with each other through the shifting of weight and turning movements.

48

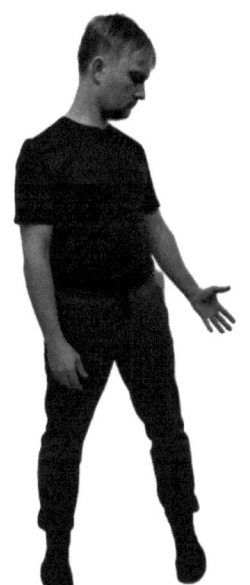

Figure 16

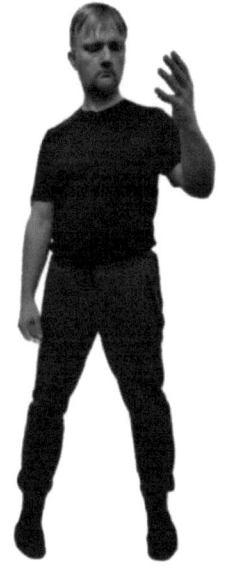

Figure 17

Summary – The 8 Golden Rules of the Qi Gong Diet

Finally, we want to summarize the knowledge about Qi Gong and Traditional Chinese Medicine that we have described in this book. The historical Buddha Sidartha Gautama called the core of his teaching the "Noble Eightfold Path". In Daoism, the "8 trigrams" from the *I Ching* (Book of Changes) represent an important symbolism. In general, according to the Far Eastern view, the 8 is considered a sacred number because it stands for infinity. The rules of the "Qi Gong diet" can also be broken down accordingly.

1. Listen to your body and follow your intuition. If your stomach tells you that you are hungry, then you should breastfeed it. If you don't feel hungry, i.e. don't feel a need for energy, then avoid consuming excess calories, e.g. through sweetened drinks and snacks.

2. Eat your meals at regular times so your metabolism can get used to them. If possible, use the Organ clock as a guide, which states that your digestive system works better in the morning and midday than later in the day.

3. When preparing your meals, make sure you give it time and leisure. Meals should be taken with pleasure and in a harmonious atmosphere. In this regard, avoid everything that has to do with stress.

4. Observe the 70% rule of Qi Gong when eating. In this context, this means that you should stop eating when you feel full. Under no circumstances should you stuff yourself to the maximum capacity.

5.Ensure that meals are balanced, i.e. most ingredients are neutral according to TCM and are not very wet, very dry, very hot or very cold. In addition, all 5 five tastes – sour, bitter, pungent, sweet, salty – should be present. In general, use as many fresh, seasonal ingredients as possible.

6.After you eat, pay close attention to how you feel afterward to find out which foods are good for you and which aren't. If, for example, you notice nausea, stomach problems or fatigue, this is an indication that your body is having problems absorbing, processing or digesting the food. Everyone is unique - find the right one for you.

7.Drink primarily tap water and herbal teas. The body needs enough liquid during the day. Immediately before or with meals, i.e. when you feel hungry, you should only drink moderately.

8.Practice Qi Gong - preferably in a daily routine. Find exercises that you enjoy and that leave you feeling energized and balanced. The smooth movements, the slow breathing and the right ideas help you to perceive yourself, to process superfluous energy reserves better and to live happier.

Overview of the practical content of the series

Jin Dao - Stay young with Qi Gong!

Volume 1: The 8 Brocades while standing and the 3 swing exercises

Volume 2: The 18 Tai Chi exercises

Volume 3: The Lohan-Qi Gong

Volume 4: The 8 Brocades while sitting and the small Heavenly circuit

Volume 5: Daoist circle walking and the Game of the 5 animals

Volume 6: Bone Marrow Qi Gong and Embryo Breathing.

Jin Dao – The Qi Gong Diet: Nutrition and movement according to TCM